Roots Apart: Navigating Life When Children Settle Abroad

C. P. Kumar
Reiki Healer
Roorkee - 247667, India

Copyright © 2023 C. P. Kumar

All rights reserved.

No part of this book may be reproduced or transmitted in any form or by any means, electronic or mechanical, including photocopying, recording, or by any information storage and retrieval system, without permission in writing from the author.

Disclaimer

While every effort has been made to ensure the accuracy and completeness of the content in this book, the author cannot guarantee that the information contained herein is error-free, up-to-date, or suitable for every individual circumstance.

The author shall not be held liable or responsible for any errors or omissions in the content of the book, nor for any damages, or losses that may arise from any actions taken based upon the suggestions or contents presented in the book.

Readers are advised to use their own judgment and discretion in applying the information provided in this book, and to consult with qualified professionals before taking any action based on the contents of this book. The author disclaims any and all liability or responsibility for any actions taken or not taken based on the information contained in this book.

DEDICATION

To all the parents who have ever watched their children spread their wings and venture far from home, this book is dedicated to you. Your love knows no borders, and your unwavering support has carried your children through uncharted territories and unknown cultures.

To the mothers and fathers who have shed countless tears, both of joy and longing, as they witness their children's growth from a distance, your strength and resilience inspire us all. Your sacrifices and selflessness are the foundations upon which your children build their futures.

To the families who have bridged the gaps of time zones and language barriers, embracing technology and cherishing every virtual connection, this dedication is for you. Your determination to stay connected, to share in the highs and lows, and to never let distance dim the flame of love is a testament to the unbreakable bonds of family.

To the children who have bravely set forth on a path of their own, leaving behind the familiar comforts of home and the embrace of loved ones, this book honors your courage and spirit of adventure. Your journey is not only one of self-discovery but also a testament to the deep-rooted values and teachings bestowed upon you.

May the pages of this book serve as a guiding light for all families navigating the complexities of life when children settle abroad. May it provide solace, wisdom, and practical insights to ease the challenges and celebrate the triumphs. Let it be a reminder that distance may separate us physically, but love transcends all borders, holding us together in heart and spirit.

With heartfelt gratitude and admiration,

C. P. Kumar

CONTENTS

PREFACE

In an increasingly interconnected world, the phenomenon of children settling abroad has become a significant part of contemporary life. The decision to migrate often brings new opportunities and adventures for the younger generation, but it also leaves behind a trail of emotions and challenges for their aging parents. As the world undergoes rapid globalization and changing family dynamics, it is essential to shed light on the experiences of elderly parents left behind and provide guidance on how to navigate the complexities of life in this new reality.

"Roots Apart: Navigating Life When Children Settle Abroad" is a comprehensive exploration of the multifaceted journey faced by aging parents who find themselves separated from their adult children. This book aims to provide insights, support, and practical advice for parents who are confronted with the unique emotional, social, financial, and healthcare challenges that arise in such circumstances.

The chapters in this book have been carefully curated to address the various aspects of life that are affected when children settle abroad. Each chapter delves into a specific theme, offering a deep understanding of the issues at hand and providing strategies for coping, adapting, and finding resilience. From the emotional impact of separation and the challenges of long-distance communication to the financial struggles, health concerns, and loss of independence, this book covers a wide range of topics relevant to the lives of aging parents.

We also explore the social and cultural implications of children settling abroad, examining the changing roles and responsibilities within the family structure and the impact of cultural and language barriers. Furthermore, we discuss the legal and administrative challenges faced by aging parents, as well as the importance of intergenerational relationships and the role of long-distance caregiving.

Throughout this book, we emphasize the significance of support systems and resources available to aging parents. We highlight the importance of building resilience, seeking therapy and support when needed, and cultivating meaningful connections within local communities. Additionally, we provide insights into the joy and complexities of reunions between adult children and their elderly parents, and offer guidance on readjusting family dynamics and managing the challenges of reverse culture shock.

In addition, two chapters in this book, 'Cultural and Language Barriers' and 'Support Systems and Resources,' also delve into the situation when children take their parents with them to settle in another country. These chapters explore the unique dynamics, adjustments, and support systems that are essential for aging parents as they embark on this journey with their adult children, shedding light on the complexities that arise in such circumstances.

"Roots Apart: Navigating Life When Children Settle Abroad" is not only a guidebook but also a testament to the strength and resilience of aging parents who face the trials of separation. It serves as a source of inspiration, reassurance, and practical knowledge for those embarking on this journey. By sharing experiences, providing guidance, and fostering empathy, we hope to assist aging parents in maintaining fulfilling lives, despite the physical distance that separates them from their children.

This book is intended for aging parents, adult children considering migration, professionals in the fields of healthcare, social work, and psychology, and anyone interested in understanding the complexities of life when children settle abroad. It is our hope that "Roots Apart" will serve as a guiding light, illuminating the path for families navigating the challenges of separation and offering a beacon of hope for a more connected and supportive future.

Remember, even when roots are physically apart, the bonds of love and family endure.

C. P. Kumar
Reiki Healer
Former Scientist 'G', National Institute of Hydrology
Roorkee - 247667, India
E-mail: cpkumar@yahoo.com
Web: https://www.angelfire.com/nh/cpkumar/virgo.html

Introduction

The phenomenon of children settling abroad has become increasingly prevalent in recent years, reshaping the dynamics of families across the globe. As children venture far from their home countries in pursuit of education, career opportunities, and personal growth, their aging parents are left to navigate a new reality filled with emotions, challenges, and uncertainties. In this book, titled "*Roots Apart: Navigating Life When Children Settle Abroad*," we delve into the experiences of aging parents who find themselves separated from their emigrant children, exploring the impact it has on their lives and providing insights and strategies to navigate this uncharted territory.

Exploring the Phenomenon of Children Settling Abroad

Migration has been an integral part of human history, with individuals and families seeking new opportunities and better lives in foreign lands. In recent decades, however, a new phenomenon has emerged – children settling abroad. This book, titled "*Roots Apart: Navigating Life When Children Settle Abroad*," delves into the unique experiences and challenges faced by aging parents when their children decide to make a permanent home in a foreign country.

The decision of children to settle abroad is often driven by a myriad of factors such as education, career prospects, economic opportunities, or personal relationships. As globalization continues to shape our world, geographic boundaries are becoming less restrictive, enabling greater mobility. Consequently, an increasing number of young adults are venturing beyond their home countries to build their lives in foreign lands.

The Impact on Aging Parents

While the decision of children to settle abroad may be a testament to their ambition and drive, it is not without consequences for their aging parents. The emotional, psychological, and practical implications for parents left behind are profound. The physical distance that separates parents and their emigrant children can create a sense of emptiness, loss, and longing. The absence of day-to-day interaction and the inability to share in the joys and challenges of their children's lives can lead to feelings of loneliness and isolation.

Furthermore, aging parents may face increased dependency on their settled children for support and care as they enter their twilight years. The traditional role reversal, where parents become dependent on their children for emotional and financial support, can be further magnified when geographical distance is added to the equation. The practical challenges of managing health issues, navigating complex bureaucracies, and maintaining a support system become more daunting for parents when their children are thousands of miles away.

Historical Context and Changing Family Dynamics in the Context of Migration

To understand the full impact of children settling abroad on aging parents, it is essential to examine the historical context and changing family dynamics associated with migration. Throughout history, migration has been a powerful force, shaping societies and transforming family structures. In earlier times, migration was often a collective endeavor, with entire families or communities uprooting themselves and resettling together in a new land.

However, the modern phenomenon of children settling abroad has introduced a new dynamic within families. It represents a departure from the traditional family unit, where generations would typically remain close and provide mutual support. The changing family dynamics associated with migration reflect a shift from the interdependence of family members to a more independent and individualistic approach to life.

The rapid advancement of technology, particularly in the realm of communication, has facilitated a level of connectivity that was unimaginable in previous eras. While parents and children may be physically separated, they can now maintain regular contact through video calls, social media platforms, and instant messaging. Despite these technological advancements, the absence of physical presence and the nuances that come with face-to-face interaction cannot be fully replaced.

Moreover, as migration becomes more common and accepted, societal norms and expectations surrounding familial obligations may evolve. The stigma or guilt associated with leaving one's parents behind in pursuit of personal aspirations may diminish. This changing landscape adds complexity to the experiences of both parents and their emigrant children as they navigate their roles and responsibilities within the context of migration.

Conclusion

This introductory chapter has set the stage for our exploration of the challenges faced by aging parents when their children settle abroad. We have examined the phenomenon of children settling abroad, the impact on aging parents, and the historical context and changing family dynamics associated with migration. Throughout this book, we will delve deeper into the emotions, experiences, and strategies that can help parents and families navigate this unique and often complex journey.

Chapter 2. Emotions and Mental Health

Introduction

When children settle abroad, embarking on new lives in foreign lands, they undoubtedly open up exciting opportunities and experiences for themselves. However, while they embark on their new journey, their elderly parents are often left behind in their home country. This separation can have a profound emotional impact on the aging parents, giving rise to a range of emotions and affecting their mental health. In this chapter, we will explore the emotional challenges faced by elderly parents when their children settle abroad, focusing on loneliness, depression, and anxiety. Additionally, we will discuss coping strategies and support systems that can help maintain their mental well-being during this period of transition.

The Emotional Impact of Separation on Elderly Parents

The separation from their children can trigger a whirlwind of emotions for elderly parents. The feeling of loss and emptiness can be overwhelming as they adjust to the absence of their children's physical presence in their daily lives. These parents have spent years nurturing and caring for their children, and suddenly finding themselves apart can leave them feeling bereft and disoriented. The emotional impact can be particularly intense if the children have settled in a country that is geographically distant, leading to limited opportunities for face-to-face communication or visits.

Loneliness, Depression, and Anxiety Among Aging Parents Left Behind

Loneliness often becomes a constant companion for elderly parents when their children settle abroad. They may feel isolated and disconnected from their social networks, as their social circles often revolved around family ties. The loss of regular interaction with their children, combined with a potential reduction in social activities, can exacerbate feelings of loneliness. This prolonged loneliness can contribute to the development of depression and anxiety disorders among aging parents.

Depression is characterized by persistent feelings of sadness, hopelessness, and a lack of interest or pleasure in activities. Elderly parents may experience a profound sense of grief over the separation from their children, leading to the onset or worsening of depressive symptoms. Anxiety, on the other hand, may manifest as excessive worry, restlessness, and a constant sense of unease. The uncertainty about their children's well-being and the challenges of navigating life without them can contribute to anxiety symptoms.

Coping Strategies and Support Systems for Maintaining Mental Well-being

While the emotional challenges faced by elderly parents are significant, there are various coping strategies and support systems that can help them maintain their mental well-being during this transitional phase.

Establishing regular communication: Maintaining regular communication with their children can provide emotional solace to aging parents. Modern technology offers numerous communication channels, such as video calls and messaging apps, allowing for more frequent and meaningful connections despite the physical distance. Encouraging children to reach out consistently and providing instructions on how to use these technologies can help bridge the gap and alleviate feelings of isolation.

Building social connections: Encouraging elderly parents to engage in social activities within their community can help combat loneliness. Joining local clubs, participating in hobby groups, or volunteering not only provides opportunities for social interaction but also enables them to form new friendships and support networks. Additionally, reaching out to other parents in similar situations can create a sense of solidarity and understanding.

Seeking professional help: If elderly parents experience persistent symptoms of depression or anxiety, it is crucial to encourage them to seek professional help. Mental health professionals, such as therapists or counselors, can provide a safe and supportive environment for parents to express their emotions and learn coping mechanisms. Therapy can help them develop resilience and navigate the challenges associated with their children settling abroad.

Engaging in self-care activities: Encouraging aging parents to prioritize self-care is essential for maintaining their mental well-being. Engaging in activities they enjoy, such as pursuing hobbies, practicing mindfulness or meditation, and maintaining a healthy lifestyle, can contribute to a more positive emotional state. Providing resources and information about self-care practices tailored to their specific needs can empower elderly parents to take care of themselves.

Conclusion

The emotional impact of separation on elderly parents when their children settle abroad should not be underestimated. Loneliness, depression, and anxiety can become significant challenges for these parents, affecting their overall mental health and well-being. However, by implementing coping strategies and accessing appropriate support systems, such as regular communication, building social connections, seeking professional help, and engaging in self-care activities, elderly parents can navigate this period of transition with greater resilience and improved mental well-being. It is crucial for both children and parents to acknowledge and address these emotional challenges, fostering open communication and understanding as they navigate life apart.

Introduction

In today's interconnected world, families often find themselves separated by vast distances as children settle abroad. This physical separation presents numerous communication challenges that must be navigated in order to maintain strong relationships. The chapter explores the complexities of long-distance communication with adult children settled in foreign lands, addresses the technological barriers that hinder effective communication, emphasizes the importance of regular and meaningful interaction, and concludes with valuable insights for families facing similar situations.

Navigating Long-Distance Communication with Adult Children Abroad

When children settle abroad, whether for education, career opportunities, or personal reasons, parents often experience a sense of longing and concern. The physical distance can create emotional gaps and communication obstacles that must be overcome. Parents may struggle to adapt to the time zone differences, and cultural nuances that shape their interactions with their children. Additionally, the limited opportunities for face-to-face communication can make it challenging to maintain a strong connection.

Technological Barriers and Solutions for Effective Communication

While technology has undoubtedly made long-distance communication more accessible, it also brings its own set of challenges. Technological barriers such as poor internet connectivity, and limited access to communication platforms can hinder effective communication.

To overcome these barriers, it is crucial for both parents and children to stay updated with the latest communication tools and platforms. Regular communication channels like email, instant messaging applications, and video calls have become indispensable for maintaining relationships across borders. Encouraging parents to learn and adapt to these technological advancements can greatly enhance their ability to connect with their children abroad.

The Importance of Regular and Meaningful Communication in Maintaining Relationships

Regular and meaningful communication plays a pivotal role in maintaining relationships between parents and their children settled abroad. It allows parents to stay informed about their children's lives, support them through challenges, and share in their successes. Similarly, children gain a sense of belonging, knowing that their parents are invested in their well-being, even from afar.

Setting up a consistent communication routine is vital. Establishing a mutually agreed-upon schedule for regular calls or video chats ensures that both parties can anticipate and prioritize their conversations. Moreover, finding the right balance between discussing practical matters, such as finances or logistics, and engaging in meaningful conversations about personal experiences and emotions is crucial for building strong bonds.

Cultivating active listening skills is equally important. Parents should create a safe space for their children to share their joys and struggles, listening attentively and offering support and guidance when needed. On the other hand, children should also make an effort to understand their parents' concerns and share their own experiences, fostering empathy and understanding between both generations.

Conclusion

Communication challenges arise when children settle abroad, disrupting the traditional dynamics of family relationships. However, with perseverance, adaptation, and the effective use of technology, these challenges can be overcome. Regular and meaningful communication acts as the bridge that connects families across borders, nurturing bonds and providing emotional support. By staying up-to-date with communication tools, establishing a consistent routine, and cultivating active listening skills, parents and children can navigate the complexities of long-distance communication and strengthen their connections.

Introduction

When children settle abroad, they embark on a journey of new opportunities and experiences. However, as they carve out their lives in a foreign land, their absence leaves a void in the lives of their aging parents back home. Beyond the emotional challenges of being separated from their children, parents often face significant financial struggles when their children settle abroad. In this chapter, we will explore the economic implications for aging parents without adequate support, the challenges of managing finances and planning for retirement in the absence of children's assistance, and the reliance on limited resources and social security systems in the country of residence.

Economic Implications for Aging Parents without Adequate Support

For many parents, the financial implications of their children settling abroad can be profound. They may have relied on their children for emotional and financial support in their old age, and without this assistance, they may find themselves facing a precarious financial situation. The absence of children often means a loss of financial contributions that would have helped cover expenses such as medical bills, housing costs, and daily necessities. This sudden shift in financial dynamics can leave aging parents vulnerable and struggling to make ends meet.

Managing Finances and Planning for Retirement in the Absence of Children's Assistance

The absence of children's assistance can have a significant impact on parents' ability to manage their finances and plan for retirement. Without the support of their children, parents may find it challenging to save enough money for their retirement years. They may have to rely solely on their own income and savings, which may be limited or insufficient to sustain a comfortable lifestyle. The burden of financial planning and ensuring a secure future falls solely on the parents' shoulders, adding stress and uncertainty to their lives.

Relying on Limited Resources and Social Security Systems in the Country of Residence

In the absence of their children's financial support, aging parents often have to rely on limited resources and the social security systems available in their country of residence. However, this can present its own set of challenges. Depending on the country, the social security benefits may be inadequate to cover the rising costs of healthcare, housing, and other essential expenses. The parents may find themselves navigating complex bureaucracies and struggling to access the support they need.

Conclusion

Financial struggles are an unfortunate reality for many aging parents when their children settle abroad. The absence of children's financial contributions can leave parents in a vulnerable position, with limited resources and increased uncertainty about their financial future. It is crucial for parents to explore alternative strategies for managing their finances, such as seeking advice from financial professionals, exploring local support systems, and making prudent financial decisions. Additionally, communities and support networks can play a vital role in providing emotional and practical assistance to parents facing financial challenges. By acknowledging the difficulties faced by aging parents and offering support and guidance, we can help bridge the gap and navigate the financial struggles that arise when children settle abroad.

Introduction

When children settle abroad, a new chapter unfolds in the lives of their parents back home. As the distance widens, so does the concern for their well-being, particularly when it comes to health and medical care. Aging brings its own set of challenges, and without the physical presence of their children, elderly parents face additional obstacles in accessing healthcare and managing their health conditions. This chapter explores the aging-related health issues, the challenges faced by elderly parents, the availability of healthcare and caregiving support, as well as strategies for managing chronic conditions and emergencies with limited local assistance.

Aging-Related Health Issues and Challenges Faced by Elderly Parents

The natural progression of age often leads to an increased risk of health issues. Elderly parents may find themselves grappling with chronic conditions such as diabetes, hypertension, arthritis, or heart disease. Additionally, age-related ailments such as osteoporosis, dementia, and vision or hearing impairment become more prevalent. These health challenges can significantly impact their daily lives and require ongoing medical attention and support.

One of the most significant challenges faced by elderly parents when children settle abroad is the emotional toll caused by the absence of their children's physical presence. The sense of security and reassurance that comes from having family members nearby during health emergencies or hospital stays can be greatly missed. The distance can lead to feelings of isolation, vulnerability, and increased anxiety.

Access to Healthcare and Caregiving Support in the Absence of Children

Accessing healthcare becomes a crucial concern for elderly parents when children settle abroad. The healthcare systems, medical practices, and cultural norms may differ between countries, making it challenging for parents to navigate the unfamiliar territory.

In the absence of their children, elderly parents may face difficulties in managing appointments, understanding medical instructions, and coordinating healthcare services. The need for an advocate or a trusted individual who can accompany them to medical appointments becomes even more critical. Navigating insurance processes and understanding healthcare costs can also be daunting tasks for elderly parents who are not familiar with the systems in place.

Moreover, the lack of informal caregiving support, which children often provide, can be particularly challenging for elderly parents. Daily tasks such as grocery shopping, meal preparation, and housekeeping may become more burdensome. The absence of emotional support and companionship from their children can also contribute to feelings of loneliness and affect their overall well-being.

Managing Chronic Conditions and Emergencies with Limited Local Support

Coping with chronic conditions can be demanding, and the absence of children can make it even more challenging for elderly parents to manage their health effectively. Adhering to medication schedules, following dietary restrictions, and maintaining an active lifestyle become tasks that require self-motivation and discipline. In the absence of familial support, staying motivated can be difficult, leading to potential health complications.

Furthermore, emergencies can arise unexpectedly, and the absence of immediate local support can cause significant stress. Elderly parents may face difficulties in seeking timely medical attention during emergencies, which can jeopardize their well-being. Establishing a network of local contacts, such as neighbors or friends, who can be relied upon in times of need becomes crucial. Creating an emergency plan that includes important medical information, contact details of local healthcare providers, and an understanding of local emergency services can help mitigate potential risks.

Conclusion

The challenges related to health and medical care that elderly parents face when children settle abroad are significant. From aging-related health issues to accessing healthcare and managing chronic conditions, the absence of children can intensify the difficulties associated with growing older. However, with proper planning, support systems, and proactive strategies, it is possible to navigate these challenges successfully.

Establishing open lines of communication with healthcare providers, engaging local support networks, and empowering elderly parents with knowledge about healthcare systems can help bridge the gap created by geographical distance. Encouraging regular health check-ups, exploring technological solutions for remote monitoring, and maintaining a strong emotional connection through frequent communication can contribute to the overall well-being of elderly parents.

Although physical proximity cannot be replaced, the love, care, and concern of children settling abroad can still be felt through constant communication, support, and ensuring that necessary arrangements are in place for the health and medical care of elderly parents. By taking these steps, families can navigate the complexities of health and medical care, finding ways to bridge the distance and ensure the well-being of their loved ones.

Introduction

As parents, we spend a significant portion of our lives nurturing and guiding our children. We invest our time, energy, and love to ensure their well-being and success. However, as they grow older, there comes a time when they embark on their own journeys, sometimes settling abroad in pursuit of new opportunities. While their pursuit of happiness is a cause for celebration, it can also lead to a profound loss of independence for parents left behind. In this chapter, we will delve into the challenges faced by parents when their children settle abroad and explore ways to navigate the difficult terrain of limited mobility, self-sufficiency, and maintaining a sense of autonomy in the face of changing circumstances.

Adjusting to a New Reality of Limited Mobility and Self-Sufficiency

When children settle abroad, parents often find themselves grappling with a new reality where their physical mobility and self-sufficiency become limited. The tasks and errands that were once effortlessly managed become daunting without the support of their children. Simple activities like grocery shopping, household repairs, and even medical appointments can become burdensome. Adjusting to this new reality requires a shift in mindset and a willingness to adapt.

One option for overcoming the challenges of limited mobility is to seek assistance from community organizations, neighbors, or friends. Many communities have programs in place that provide support and services to elderly individuals. These programs can include transportation services, home-delivered meals, and even assistance with household chores. By reaching out and embracing these resources, parents can regain a sense of control over their daily lives.

Exploring Options for Assisted Living and Elderly Care in the Absence of Children

In some cases, the loss of independence can be more pronounced, necessitating a consideration of assisted living or elderly care options. The prospect of leaving the comfort of one's home and moving into an assisted living facility can be overwhelming. However, it is essential to remember that such facilities are designed to provide the care and support needed to ensure a high quality of life for older adults.

Before making any decisions, it is crucial for parents to thoroughly research and visit various assisted living facilities or explore home care options. It is essential to consider factors such as the staff-to-resident ratio, the range of services provided, the overall atmosphere of the facility, and the cost involved. By actively participating in the decision-making process, parents can maintain a sense of control over their lives and ensure that their needs and preferences are met.

Maintaining a Sense of Autonomy and Independence Despite the Circumstances

While the physical aspects of independence may diminish with age and the absence of children, it is vital for parents to nurture their emotional and psychological independence. This can be achieved through various means:

Cultivating Hobbies and Interests: Engaging in activities that bring joy and fulfillment can help parents maintain a sense of purpose and individuality. Whether it's painting, gardening, reading, or joining clubs or community groups, exploring new passions can foster a sense of independence and personal growth.

Building a Support Network: Establishing connections with peers, neighbors, and friends is crucial for combatting feelings of isolation and dependence. Regular social interactions can provide emotional support and a sense of belonging, reminding parents that they are not alone in their journey.

Embracing Technology: The digital age offers a multitude of opportunities for maintaining independence and staying connected with loved ones. Learning to use smartphones, video chat applications, and social media platforms can bridge the geographical gap between parents and their children, fostering a sense of closeness and involvement in their lives.

Conclusion

The loss of independence experienced by parents when their children settle abroad can be a challenging and emotional journey. Adjusting to limited mobility, exploring assisted living options, and maintaining a sense of autonomy requires resilience, adaptability, and a proactive approach. By embracing community resources, considering assisted living or home care options, and nurturing emotional and psychological independence, parents can navigate this chapter of their lives with grace and dignity. While the physical distance may separate them from their children, it doesn't have to diminish the richness and fulfillment of their own lives. Remember, even in the face of change, independence can be redefined and rediscovered.

Introduction

In the age of globalization, the phenomenon of children settling abroad has become increasingly common. While this offers numerous opportunities and benefits for the younger generation, it often leads to significant challenges for the elderly parents who are left behind in their home country. One such challenge is social isolation, which can have profound effects on the well-being of aging parents. In this chapter, we will explore the impact of social isolation on the well-being of elderly parents left behind, discuss the importance of social connections and community engagement for them, and provide strategies for creating opportunities for social interaction and meaningful relationships within the local community.

Impact of Social Isolation on the Well-being of Elderly Parents Left Behind

Social isolation can be detrimental to the physical, emotional, and mental well-being of elderly parents. When children settle abroad, parents often experience a significant decrease in social interaction and support networks. They may feel lonely, disconnected, and neglected, leading to feelings of sadness, depression, and anxiety. Lack of social engagement can also lead to physical health issues as it may result in a sedentary lifestyle and decreased motivation for self-care. Without regular social interactions, elderly parents may experience a decline in cognitive function and a diminished sense of purpose in life. All of these factors combined can contribute to a lower quality of life for aging parents.

Importance of Social Connections and Community Engagement for Aging Parents

Maintaining social connections and engaging with the local community is crucial for the well-being of aging parents. Social interactions provide emotional support, a sense of belonging, and opportunities for companionship. They also play a vital role in preserving cognitive function and mental well-being. Being part of a community helps elderly parents feel valued, respected, and included, which in turn boosts their self-esteem and overall happiness. Regular engagement in social activities can also improve physical health by promoting an active lifestyle and reducing the risk of certain health conditions. Moreover, social connections create opportunities for personal growth, learning, and the development of new skills.

Creating Opportunities for Social Interaction and Meaningful Relationships within the Local Community

To combat social isolation and promote a fulfilling life for elderly parents left behind, it is important to create opportunities for social interaction and meaningful relationships within the local community. Here are some strategies that can be implemented:

Establish Community Programs: Encourage the development of community programs specifically tailored to the needs and interests of aging parents. These programs can include social clubs, hobby groups, and support networks. Local community centers, religious institutions, and senior centers are excellent starting points for finding such initiatives.

Volunteer Activities: Encourage elderly parents to engage in volunteer work. Volunteering not only provides an opportunity for social interaction but also enables them to contribute to society and feel a sense of purpose. They can explore organizations that align with their interests and skills, such as libraries, hospitals, animal shelters, or charities.

Participate in Local Events: Encourage elderly parents to participate in local events, festivals, and cultural activities. This allows them to experience the richness of their community, connect with others, and celebrate their heritage. Local newspapers, community notice boards, and online platforms can provide information about upcoming events.

Digital Connectivity: Teach elderly parents how to use technology to stay connected with their children abroad, as well as with local friends and family. Social media platforms, video calls, and messaging apps can bridge the geographical gap and provide regular communication and emotional support.

Support Groups: Encourage elderly parents to join support groups or counseling sessions specifically designed for individuals who are dealing with the challenges of their children settling abroad. These groups can provide a safe space for sharing experiences, emotions, and coping strategies.

Intergenerational Programs: Promote intergenerational programs that bring together elderly parents and younger generations. This can include mentorship programs, intergenerational learning initiatives, or partnerships with schools and universities. Interacting with younger individuals can provide a sense of purpose, foster learning, and create meaningful relationships.

Conclusion

Social isolation poses significant challenges for elderly parents left behind when their children settle abroad. It affects their physical health, emotional well-being, and overall quality of life. However, by recognizing the importance of social connections and community engagement, we can mitigate the negative effects of social isolation. Creating opportunities for social interaction and meaningful relationships within the local community is crucial. Through community programs, volunteer activities, participation in local events, digital connectivity, support groups, and intergenerational programs, we can help aging parents combat social isolation and navigate their lives with a sense of purpose, belonging, and fulfillment. It is through these efforts that we can bridge the gap between generations and nurture stronger bonds within families, regardless of geographical distance.

Chapter 8. Changing Roles and Responsibilities

Introduction

In today's globalized world, the phenomenon of children settling abroad has become increasingly common. As the younger generation ventures out to pursue education, career opportunities, or personal aspirations in foreign lands, families are faced with significant changes in their dynamics and relationships. The once familiar family structure is reshaped, and as a result, roles and responsibilities undergo a transformation. This chapter delves into the intricacies of these changes and explores the challenges and opportunities that arise when children settle abroad.

Shifting Dynamics within the Family Structure due to Children Settling Abroad

When children settle abroad, the dynamics within the family structure inevitably undergo a profound shift. Traditionally, parents have assumed the roles of caregivers, providers, and decision-makers, guiding their children through various stages of life. However, with the physical distance created by emigration, the balance of power and influence often undergoes a transformation. Children who settle abroad gain independence, take on new responsibilities, and become more self-reliant. This can lead to a redistribution of roles within the family.

Role Reversal between Parents and Children in Terms of Caregiving and Support

One significant aspect of changing roles and responsibilities is the role reversal that may occur between parents and their children. In many cultures, it is customary for adult children to take care of their aging parents. However, when children settle abroad, this dynamic can be reversed. Parents may find themselves needing support and care as they grow older, while their children, despite being physically distant, are expected to provide emotional and financial support. This reversal can be emotionally challenging for both parents and children, as it requires adapting to new expectations and redefining the meaning of filial duty.

Redefining Expectations, Boundaries, and Family Roles in the Absence of Children

The absence of children due to settlement abroad also necessitates a reevaluation of expectations, boundaries, and family roles. Parents may have envisioned a future where their children would continue to live nearby, provide support, and eventually take over certain responsibilities. However, with children living far away, parents may need to readjust their expectations and find new sources of support and companionship within their local community or extended family. Similarly, children settling abroad may need to redefine their roles within the family, considering their limited physical presence and the challenges of managing familial responsibilities from afar.

Communication and technology play crucial roles in maintaining connections and bridging the physical gap. Video calls, messaging apps, and social media platforms have made it easier for families to stay in touch and share experiences. However, the reliance on technology can also lead to emotional challenges, as virtual interactions may not fully substitute for physical presence. Striking a balance between maintaining connections and respecting individual boundaries becomes essential.

Conclusion

The process of children settling abroad brings about a myriad of changes within the family unit. Roles and responsibilities shift, and a redefinition of expectations and boundaries becomes necessary. Parents may find themselves relying on their children for support, both emotionally and financially, despite the physical distance. Likewise, adult children must navigate the complexities of providing care and maintaining relationships from afar. While these changes can be challenging, they also present opportunities for growth, resilience, and a deepening of family bonds.

Navigating changing roles and responsibilities requires open and honest communication, understanding, and flexibility from all family members. It is essential to acknowledge and address any emotional challenges that arise during this transition, seeking support from friends, professionals, or support groups when needed. Embracing the new dynamics and redefining family roles can lead to strengthened relationships and a deeper understanding of the complexities of modern family life in a globalized world.

Ultimately, the journey of navigating life when children settle abroad is an ongoing process of adaptation and growth. By embracing these changes and finding new ways to connect and support one another, families can bridge the physical distance and thrive amidst the challenges and opportunities that arise.

Introduction

When children settle abroad, whether for education, work, or personal reasons, they embark on a journey that often spans generations and countries. This journey not only affects the children themselves but also their elders, especially when they decide to take their parents with them to settle in another country. While this adventure brings new opportunities and experiences, it also presents challenges, particularly for elderly parents who may find themselves in an unfamiliar cultural and linguistic environment. One of the most significant obstacles they face is navigating these cultural and language barriers. In this chapter, we will explore the profound impact of these barriers on both elderly parents and their migrant children, and discuss strategies for bridging the gap to foster understanding and support.

Cultural Differences Between Generations and Countries Affecting Elderly Parents

Cultural differences between generations and countries can be a source of both excitement and tension. Elderly parents who have spent their lives in a particular cultural context may find it challenging to adapt to the customs, values, and social norms of their children's adopted country. They may struggle to understand the new societal structures, traditions, and expectations that differ from their own. These disparities can lead to feelings of isolation, confusion, and even resentment.

Moreover, the generation gap adds another layer of complexity to the cultural divide. The children who settle

41

abroad often embrace their host country's culture more readily, influenced by their surroundings and peers. This can create a disconnection between parents and children, as their beliefs and perspectives may clash due to differing cultural influences. The elderly parents may feel alienated from their children's lives, further exacerbating their sense of displacement and detachment.

Language Barriers and Their Impact on Integration and Support for Aging Parents

Language is the cornerstone of communication and understanding. For elderly parents who do not speak the language of their children's adopted country, language barriers pose significant challenges. Limited language proficiency hampers their ability to integrate into the local community, engage in social interactions, access services, and navigate daily life. This isolation can lead to feelings of frustration, loneliness, and dependency on their children for even the most basic tasks.

Language barriers also hinder the provision of adequate support for aging parents. Miscommunication or a lack of understanding can make it difficult for children to meet their parents' needs, whether it is seeking appropriate healthcare, arranging social activities, or addressing legal and financial matters. The inability to effectively communicate may result in misunderstandings, strained relationships, and a sense of powerlessness for both parties involved.

Bridging the Cultural and Linguistic Gap to Foster Understanding and Support

Recognizing the significance of cultural and language barriers, it is crucial to adopt strategies that bridge the gap and promote understanding and support. Here are some approaches that can help facilitate this process:

Cultural Exchange and Education: Encourage open and respectful dialogue between generations. Both parents and children should be willing to learn from each other's cultural perspectives, beliefs, and values. Organizing family gatherings, cultural events, or sharing stories and traditions can foster mutual understanding and strengthen bonds.

Language Learning: Encourage elderly parents to learn the language of their children's adopted country. Language classes, community language programs, or even language exchange initiatives can provide opportunities for them to improve their language skills. Children can also take on the role of language facilitators, assisting their parents in practicing the new language.

Cultural Sensitivity and Patience: Children settling abroad should strive to be culturally sensitive and patient with their elderly parents. Recognize the challenges they face in adapting to a new environment and be understanding of their perspectives and emotions. Cultivate an environment of empathy and support.

Support Networks: Seek out local support networks, community organizations, and senior centers that cater to the needs of elderly immigrants. These networks can provide a sense of belonging, social connections, and assistance in navigating the challenges of a new culture and language.

Technology and Online Resources: Utilize technology and online resources to bridge the physical distance. Video calls, social media platforms, and translation apps can help maintain regular communication and provide a platform for sharing experiences and fostering connections.

Conclusion

Cultural and language barriers pose significant challenges for both elderly parents and their children settling abroad. The disconnect caused by these barriers can lead to feelings of isolation, frustration, and a strained parent-child relationship. However, with conscious effort and empathy, it is possible to bridge the cultural and linguistic gap and foster understanding and support. By embracing cultural exchange, language learning, patience, and support networks, families can navigate the complexities of life abroad and ensure a sense of unity and connectedness across generations and countries.

Chapter 10. Parental Expectations and Guilt

Introduction

When children settle abroad, it often marks a significant milestone in their lives. They embark on a journey to explore new opportunities, pursue higher education, or establish their careers in foreign lands. While this experience can be incredibly rewarding and transformative, it also comes with its fair share of challenges, particularly when it comes to managing parental expectations and coping with feelings of guilt. In this chapter, we will delve into the complexities of this emotional landscape and explore strategies to navigate the delicate balance between personal aspirations and obligations towards aging parents.

Managing Parental Expectations and Coping with Feelings of Guilt

When children leave their home country to settle abroad, parents may have certain expectations and dreams for their future. They envision their children leading successful lives, achieving milestones, and creating a secure and comfortable future for themselves. However, when reality unfolds differently, parents may experience a range of emotions, including disappointment, worry, and even a sense of personal failure.

As children settle abroad, it is important for both parties to acknowledge and address these expectations. Open and honest communication becomes the key to bridging the gap between parental aspirations and the realities faced by their children. Sharing experiences, discussing challenges, and expressing genuine empathy can help parents understand the unique circumstances their children encounter in a foreign land.

Equally important is for children to recognize and cope with the feelings of guilt that may arise. Guilt can stem from a sense of leaving parents behind, feeling responsible for their emotional well-being, or even for not meeting their expectations. It is crucial for children to understand that pursuing their dreams and aspirations does not invalidate the love and care they have for their parents. Acknowledging and accepting these emotions is the first step towards finding a healthy balance.

Balancing Personal Aspirations and Obligations towards Aging Parents

One of the most challenging aspects for individuals settling abroad is striking a balance between their personal aspirations and their obligations towards aging parents. As parents grow older, their needs and vulnerabilities may increase, and children often grapple with the guilt of not being physically present to support them.

In such situations, cultivating empathy becomes vital. Both children and parents must strive to understand each other's perspectives. Children can take proactive steps to ensure their parents' well-being, such as regular communication, exploring ways to provide assistance from afar, or even considering the possibility of a visit or relocation if circumstances permit.

At the same time, it is crucial for children to nurture their own growth and personal development. Pursuing dreams and seizing opportunities does not diminish the love and respect they hold for their parents. It is essential to strike a balance that allows for personal growth while also fulfilling responsibilities towards aging parents. This balance may involve seeking support from extended family members, friends, or local communities, as well as exploring available resources and services that can provide assistance to parents in need.

Cultivating Empathy, Effective Communication, and Setting Realistic Expectations

The foundation for managing parental expectations and guilt lies in cultivating empathy, fostering effective communication, and setting realistic expectations. Both children and parents must make a conscious effort to understand each other's perspectives, needs, and limitations.

Empathy is the ability to put oneself in another's shoes, to understand their emotions and experiences. Parents need to empathize with the challenges their children face in a foreign land, such as language barriers, cultural differences, and the pressures of building a new life from scratch. Similarly, children must empathize with the concerns and expectations of their parents, recognizing their desire for their children's happiness and success.

Effective communication is a powerful tool in navigating the complexities of this relationship. Regular and open dialogue helps build trust, fosters understanding, and ensures that both parties have a clear understanding of each other's desires and limitations. Children should communicate their aspirations and challenges honestly, while parents should express their concerns and expectations in a supportive manner.

Setting realistic expectations is essential for maintaining a healthy and balanced relationship. Parents and children must recognize that circumstances may differ from what they initially envisioned. Flexibility and adaptability become critical in adjusting expectations to align with the realities of settling abroad. This involves acknowledging the challenges faced by children and appreciating their efforts, even if they do not match preconceived notions of success.

Conclusion

Navigating parental expectations and guilt when children settle abroad is a delicate dance that requires understanding, empathy, and effective communication. Parents and children must embark on a journey of mutual growth, embracing the opportunities and challenges that come with living in different corners of the world. By striking a balance between personal aspirations and obligations towards aging parents, cultivating empathy, and setting realistic expectations, families can build resilient relationships that transcend physical distance. In doing so, they can create a support network that spans continents, enriching each other's lives and fostering a sense of belonging despite the roots that lie apart.

Chapter 11. Legal and Administrative Challenges

Introduction

When children settle abroad, they embark on a new journey, leaving behind their parents in their home country. This separation brings about a multitude of challenges, including legal and administrative hurdles that need to be navigated. In this chapter, we will explore the various legal and administrative challenges faced by parents when their children settle abroad and discuss potential solutions to address these issues.

Navigating Legal Systems and Documentation Requirements in the Absence of Children

One of the primary challenges faced by parents when their children settle abroad is the need to navigate unfamiliar legal systems and fulfill documentation requirements. This can be particularly daunting for elderly parents who may not be well-versed in the legal processes of the host country. Simple tasks such as signing legal documents, accessing healthcare, or managing finances may become arduous undertakings.

To overcome these challenges, it is essential for parents to seek support and guidance from local legal professionals or community organizations specializing in immigrant issues. These resources can provide valuable information on the legal requirements, assist in preparing necessary documents, and guide parents through the process. Additionally, parents can rely on their children to assist in understanding and navigating the legal systems, either by providing remote guidance or arranging for local legal representation.

Power of Attorney and Guardianship Issues for Elderly Parents

Another significant concern for children settling abroad is the question of power of attorney and guardianship for their elderly parents who remain in the home country. Parents often face dilemmas regarding decision-making authority and ensuring the well-being of their aging parents from a distance.

To address these concerns, parents should consider establishing a power of attorney arrangement with a trusted individual or a legal professional in the home country. A power of attorney grants authority to act on behalf of the elderly parents, allowing decisions to be made in their best interests. It is crucial to involve the elderly parents in discussions and ensure that their wishes and preferences are respected throughout the process.

In cases where parents anticipate the need for long-term care or guardianship for their elderly parents, it may be necessary to engage local legal counsel to navigate the specific laws and regulations governing guardianship arrangements in the host country. These legal professionals can provide guidance on the legal procedures involved and assist in establishing guardianship to ensure the well-being of the elderly parents.

Accessing Benefits and Entitlements for Elderly Parents without Local Support

When children settle abroad, their parents may face challenges in accessing benefits and entitlements they are entitled to in their home country. Navigating government systems, managing paperwork, and meeting eligibility criteria can be overwhelming for elderly parents, especially when they lack local support networks.

To overcome these challenges, parents can explore local community organizations, immigrant support groups, or senior citizen associations that offer assistance in accessing benefits and entitlements. These organizations often have staff or volunteers who are knowledgeable about the processes and can help parents navigate the administrative requirements.

Additionally, parents should encourage their elderly parents to explore resources available in their home country, such as social welfare agencies, community centers, or senior citizen programs. These local resources can provide valuable support and guidance to ensure that the elderly parents receive the benefits and entitlements they deserve.

Conclusion

The legal and administrative challenges faced by parents when their children settle abroad are significant and require careful navigation. By seeking guidance from local legal professionals, establishing power of attorney arrangements, and accessing community resources, parents can overcome these challenges and ensure the well-being of their elderly parents. It is crucial to approach these challenges proactively, involving all parties concerned and respecting the wishes and preferences of the elderly parents throughout the process. With proper planning and support, parents can effectively manage the legal and administrative complexities and successfully navigate life when children settle abroad.

Chapter 12. Intergenerational Relationships

Introduction

As the world becomes more interconnected, it is increasingly common for families to be spread across different countries and continents. This global diaspora brings with it a unique set of challenges, particularly for the older generation who find themselves separated from their children and grandchildren. However, despite the physical distance, intergenerational relationships can remain strong and meaningful. In this chapter, we explore the various ways in which families can navigate the complexities of maintaining strong bonds across generations when children settle abroad.

Strengthening Bonds Between Generations Despite the Distance

Distance may pose a challenge to maintaining strong intergenerational relationships, but it is not an insurmountable obstacle. Thanks to modern technology, staying connected with loved ones across the globe has never been easier. Video calls, messaging apps, and social media platforms provide opportunities for regular communication and virtual face-to-face interactions. Through these mediums, grandparents can witness their grandchildren's growth, share stories, and provide guidance, despite the physical separation.

Moreover, it is crucial for both parents and children to prioritize these relationships and make a conscious effort to stay connected. Scheduling regular check-ins, sharing updates about daily life, and involving grandparents in important decision-making processes can help bridge the gap and maintain a strong sense of familial connection.

Maintaining a Sense of Family and Cultural Heritage for Elderly Parents

When children settle abroad, elderly parents often face the challenge of preserving their sense of family and cultural heritage. Being away from their children and grandchildren may lead to feelings of isolation and a disconnection from their roots. To address this, it is essential for the younger generation to actively involve their parents in their new lives.

One way to accomplish this is by incorporating cultural traditions and practices into daily life, even when living in a different country. Celebrating important festivals, preparing traditional meals, and involving grandparents in decision-making regarding cultural matters can help them feel valued and connected to their heritage. Additionally, organizing trips to visit the home country, if feasible, can provide elderly parents with the opportunity to reunite with extended family, revisit familiar places, and strengthen their cultural identity.

Celebrating Milestones and Creating Shared Experiences Despite Physical Separation

Physical separation does not mean missing out on important milestones and creating shared experiences as a family. Technology once again plays a crucial role in bridging this gap. Virtual celebrations, such as birthdays, graduations, and anniversaries, can be organized, allowing grandparents to be a part of these significant events. Coordinating surprise deliveries, sending personalized messages, and engaging in shared activities through video calls can help create a sense of togetherness, despite the distance.

In addition to virtual celebrations, planning periodic visits can provide an opportunity for creating cherished memories together. Setting aside dedicated time to spend with grandparents during these visits, whether through exploring new places, engaging in shared hobbies, or simply enjoying quality time together, can strengthen the bond and provide a sense of continuity in the relationship.

Conclusion

Navigating intergenerational relationships when children settle abroad requires effort, commitment, and a willingness to adapt to the challenges posed by distance. By utilizing the available technology, maintaining a strong sense of family and cultural heritage, and actively involving elderly parents in their new lives, families can overcome the physical separation and foster meaningful connections across generations. Although the distance may present obstacles, it is possible to celebrate milestones, create shared experiences, and strengthen the bonds that tie families together. Through these efforts, families can navigate the complexities of living apart while still feeling connected, supported, and loved.

Chapter 13. Long-Distance Caregiving

Introduction

In today's globalized world, it is increasingly common for children to settle abroad, leaving their aging parents behind in their home country. This separation poses unique challenges for both the children and the parents, particularly when it comes to caregiving. Long-distance caregiving involves providing support and assistance to aging parents from afar, and it requires careful planning, effective communication, and creative solutions. In this chapter, we will explore the challenges faced by long-distance caregivers and discuss strategies to overcome them, including coordinating care and support networks from a distance and utilizing technology and local resources for remote caregiving.

Challenges Faced by Long-Distance Caregivers

Long-distance caregiving presents a range of emotional, logistical, and practical challenges. One of the primary difficulties is the emotional strain of being physically separated from loved ones who may be experiencing health issues or age-related decline. The guilt and anxiety that often accompany long-distance caregiving can take a toll on the caregiver's well-being.

Another challenge is the limited availability of information about the parent's day-to-day life and health status. Long-distance caregivers may struggle to stay informed about their parent's medical appointments, medications, and overall well-being. This lack of proximity can make it challenging to assess the situation accurately and provide appropriate support.

Coordinating Care and Support Networks from a Distance

Despite the physical distance, long-distance caregivers can play a crucial role in coordinating care and support networks for their aging parents. Effective communication becomes paramount in these situations. Regular check-ins with the parent and local caregivers, such as family members, neighbors, or friends, can provide valuable insights into the parent's well-being and any emerging needs.

Establishing open lines of communication with healthcare professionals involved in the parent's care is vital. Long-distance caregivers should request permission to receive medical updates, test results, and treatment plans directly from the healthcare providers. This way, they can stay informed about the parent's health and actively participate in decision-making.

Creating a support network for the parent is also essential. Long-distance caregivers can connect with local community organizations, senior centers, or religious institutions to identify resources that can assist their parents. These resources may include transportation services, meal delivery programs, or social activities tailored for seniors. By leveraging these local networks, long-distance caregivers can help enhance their parents' quality of life.

Utilizing Technology and Local Resources for Remote Caregiving

Advancements in technology have made long-distance caregiving more manageable. Various digital tools and platforms can bridge the gap between the caregiver and the parent, facilitating communication, monitoring, and coordination. Video calls, messaging apps, and social media platforms allow for frequent and meaningful interactions, offering a sense of closeness despite the distance.

Remote monitoring devices can also be employed to ensure the parent's safety and well-being. These devices can track vital signs, detect falls, or remind the parent to take medications. By utilizing such technology, long-distance caregivers can stay informed about their parent's health status and intervene promptly if any concerns arise.

Local resources should not be overlooked either. Researching and connecting with local support groups or caregiver organizations in the parent's community can provide valuable insights and guidance. These resources can offer practical advice, emotional support, and even connect long-distance caregivers with local volunteers who can assist in certain caregiving tasks.

Conclusion

Long-distance caregiving comes with its unique set of challenges, but with careful planning, effective communication, and the use of technology and local resources, these challenges can be overcome. It is crucial for long-distance caregivers to establish strong communication channels with their aging parents, healthcare providers, and local support networks. By staying informed, involved, and connected, long-distance caregivers can provide the necessary support and ensure their parents' well-being, even from afar. Ultimately, long-distance caregiving is a testament to the enduring bonds between parents and children, demonstrating that love and care can transcend physical distance.

Introduction

When children settle abroad, parents often find themselves navigating a new phase of life, one marked by separation and the challenges that come with it. It is during this period that coping strategies and resilience become vital tools for managing the emotional and practical aspects of life. In this chapter, we will explore the various coping strategies that can help parents build resilience, find purpose, and seek support when needed. By understanding and implementing these strategies, parents can navigate the complexities of their changing lives with strength and adaptability.

Building Resilience in the Face of Separation and Challenges for Aging Parents

The separation from children can be emotionally overwhelming for parents, especially as they age. It is crucial for parents to build resilience, which enables them to bounce back from adversity and adapt to new circumstances. One effective strategy is to maintain a positive mindset and focus on the opportunities that arise from their children's settlement abroad. Parents can develop new hobbies, pursue interests they have neglected, or engage in volunteer work. By embracing change and exploring new avenues, they can find fulfillment and purpose in their lives, independent of their children's presence.

Furthermore, establishing a support network is essential for coping with separation. Engaging with other parents who are in similar situations can provide a sense of belonging and understanding. Joining support groups, attending community events, or participating in online forums can create opportunities for shared experiences and emotional support. Additionally, maintaining open lines of communication with their children and leveraging technology can bridge the physical gap, helping parents feel connected and involved in their children's lives.

Finding Purpose and Meaning in Life Beyond the Presence of Children

Parents must navigate the shift from being actively involved in their children's lives to discovering their own purpose and meaning. This transitional period offers a chance for parents to reassess their goals and aspirations, unburdened by the immediate responsibilities of parenting. They can embark on a journey of self-discovery, exploring new interests, and rekindling old passions. Pursuing education, engaging in creative endeavors, or embarking on new careers are ways in which parents can find fulfillment and create a renewed sense of purpose.

Additionally, contributing to the community and giving back can foster a sense of meaning in life. Parents can volunteer their time and skills to local organizations, mentor younger generations, or engage in philanthropic activities. By making a positive impact on others, parents can find a sense of purpose that extends beyond their role as parents, enriching their own lives and the lives of those around them.

Seeking Support, Therapy, and Cultivating Resilience When Needed

While building resilience is crucial, it is also important to recognize when additional support is needed. Aging parents facing separation and the challenges that come with it may experience emotional distress, loneliness, or anxiety. Seeking professional help, such as therapy or counseling, can provide a safe space for parents to process their emotions and develop coping strategies. Therapists can assist in navigating the complexities of separation, offering guidance and support tailored to the unique circumstances of each individual.

Cultivating resilience also involves self-care practices. Engaging in activities that promote mental and physical well-being, such as regular exercise, meditation, and maintaining a healthy lifestyle, can significantly contribute to one's resilience. Additionally, practicing self-compassion and accepting the challenges that come with separation can help parents develop a resilient mindset, enabling them to adapt and grow stronger in the face of adversity.

Conclusion

Navigating life when children settle abroad presents a unique set of challenges for parents. However, by implementing coping strategies and cultivating resilience, parents can embrace this new phase with strength and adaptability. Building resilience allows parents to find purpose and meaning beyond the presence of their children, while seeking support and therapy ensures they have the resources necessary to navigate emotional difficulties. By leveraging these strategies, parents can not only overcome the challenges of separation but also discover new opportunities for personal growth and fulfillment.

Introduction

Reunions hold a special place in the hearts of individuals separated by time and distance. When adult children settle abroad, the anticipation of reuniting with their elderly parents is often a mix of excitement and apprehension. The journey of reunion and reintegration brings with it both joy and complexities, as families navigate the adjustments necessary to rebuild relationships and readjust their dynamics. In this chapter, we will explore the various aspects of reunions between adult children and elderly parents, highlighting the challenges posed by long separations and the process of reintegration into the family unit.

The Joy and Complexities of Reunions

Reunions between adult children and their elderly parents are often marked by an overwhelming sense of joy and relief. After months or even years of separation, the opportunity to embrace, share stories, and create new memories is cherished. The emotional bonds forged during reunions serve as a powerful reminder of the enduring connection between family members.

However, alongside the joy, there are complexities that emerge when reuniting after a long separation. Adult children may find that their parents have aged significantly since their last meeting, confronting them with the realities of mortality and the passing of time. The roles and dynamics within the family might have shifted during the separation, and both parties must navigate these changes to establish a new equilibrium.

Adjusting to Changes and Readjusting Family Dynamics

When adult children settle abroad, their lives often undergo significant transformations. They immerse themselves in new cultures, acquire new perspectives, and develop independence. Meanwhile, their parents continue their lives in their home country, adapting to the absence of their children and facing the challenges of aging.

Reunions bring together individuals who have evolved in different environments, leading to adjustments on both sides. Adult children may have grown accustomed to their newfound independence and developed unique ways of life. They may need to readjust their expectations and find a balance between honoring their heritage and embracing the changes they have undergone.

Similarly, elderly parents may have developed new routines and coping mechanisms to navigate life without their children. Their children's return can disrupt these routines and require them to adapt to new dynamics within the family. Communication and understanding become vital in renegotiating roles and finding common ground.

Challenges of Reverse Culture Shock

While reunions offer an opportunity for celebration, they can also be accompanied by challenges, particularly in cases where adult children are returning to their home country after an extended period abroad. Reverse culture shock, a phenomenon experienced by individuals readjusting to their home culture, can pose significant hurdles to successful reintegration.

Returning children may find themselves grappling with a sense of displacement, as they have become accustomed to a different way of life and have adopted new cultural norms. They may feel like strangers in their own homeland, struggling to reconcile their experiences abroad with the familiar aspects of their upbringing.

Similarly, their parents may struggle to fully comprehend the changes their children have undergone. The clash between the values and perspectives acquired abroad and the traditional expectations of their home culture can create tension and misunderstandings. Patience, empathy, and open communication are crucial in navigating the complexities of reverse culture shock and facilitating a smooth reintegration process.

Conclusion

Reunions between adult children and elderly parents offer an opportunity to bridge the gaps created by time and distance. They are marked by joy, but also present challenges as families readjust to changes and rebuild relationships. The process of reintegration requires flexibility, understanding, and a willingness to adapt to the evolving dynamics within the family.

Navigating the complexities of reunion and reintegration requires open communication, empathy, and a shared commitment to embracing both the shared heritage and the individual growth experienced by each family member. With patience and understanding, reunions can become transformative experiences that strengthen the bonds between adult children and their elderly parents, fostering a deeper connection that transcends geographical boundaries and time.

Introduction

When children settle abroad, their elderly parents often face unique challenges and uncertainties in navigating life in a new country. In this chapter, we will explore the importance of support systems and resources available to assist elderly parents in adapting to their new environment. We will delve into identifying local and international support organizations, government programs and services, as well as the significance of building a network of support and sharing experiences with others in similar situations. By harnessing these support systems and resources, we can help bridge the gap and provide a sense of stability and well-being for aging parents in their new homeland.

Identifying Local and International Support Organizations for Elderly Parents

One of the first steps in assisting elderly parents who have settled abroad is to identify local and international support organizations that can provide valuable resources and assistance. These organizations specialize in offering a range of services tailored to the needs of aging individuals. They often provide social activities, counseling, healthcare support, and educational programs designed to enhance the well-being and quality of life of elderly parents.

Local support organizations can be found through various channels, including community centers, religious institutions, and social service agencies. These organizations often have a deep understanding of the local culture and can offer personalized assistance to elderly parents, ensuring they feel connected and supported in their new surroundings.

International support organizations, on the other hand, cater specifically to expatriate communities and offer a unique perspective for elderly parents settling abroad. These organizations understand the challenges and specific needs of those who have left their home country and can provide a network of support within the expat community. They often organize social events, support groups, and language classes, fostering a sense of belonging and camaraderie among expatriate parents.

Government Programs and Services Available to Support Aging Parents

Governments worldwide recognize the importance of supporting aging parents and have implemented programs and services to address their specific needs. These programs aim to provide financial assistance, healthcare support, and social welfare benefits to elderly individuals.

Financial support programs such as pension schemes, subsidies, and tax benefits can help alleviate financial burdens for elderly parents settling abroad. These programs can provide a sense of security and stability, allowing parents to focus on their well-being and integration into the new society.

Healthcare support is another crucial aspect of government programs for aging parents. Many countries offer comprehensive healthcare coverage, including access to hospitals, clinics, and prescription medications. Additionally, specialized services for mental health, geriatric care, and home healthcare can ensure that elderly parents receive the necessary medical attention and support.

Social welfare benefits, including social security allowances, disability support, and caregiver support, can also play a vital role in helping elderly parents settle abroad. These benefits offer a safety net and assistance to those in need, promoting a sense of inclusivity and well-being within the community.

Building a Network of Support and Sharing Experiences with Others in Similar Situations

Loneliness and isolation can often be significant challenges for elderly parents settling abroad. However, by building a network of support and sharing experiences with others in similar situations, parents can find solace, companionship, and practical guidance.

Expatriate community groups, social clubs, and online forums provide platforms for elderly parents to connect with individuals who share similar backgrounds and experiences. These groups can offer valuable advice, organize social events, and provide a sense of community for parents who may feel detached from their familiar surroundings.

Furthermore, support groups specifically tailored for aging parents can create a safe space for individuals to share their concerns, exchange coping strategies, and provide emotional support. These groups often organize regular meetings, workshops, and seminars, fostering an environment of understanding and empathy.

Conclusion

Support systems and resources play a pivotal role in helping elderly parents navigate life when their children settle abroad. By identifying local and international support organizations, accessing government programs and services, and building a network of support, we can provide a sense of stability, well-being, and belonging for aging parents in their new homeland. It is through these support systems that we can bridge the gap between cultures, foster resilience, and ensure that elderly parents thrive in their new environment.

"Roots Apart: Navigating Life When Children Settle Abroad" is a comprehensive guidebook that delves into the profound challenges faced by aging parents when their children settle abroad. In this thought-provoking book, each chapter tackles a different aspect of this complex issue, providing valuable insights, practical advice, and real-life stories. From exploring the emotional impact of separation to managing financial struggles, navigating communication barriers, and addressing health and caregiving concerns, the book offers a holistic perspective on the unique circumstances faced by elderly parents left behind. It also delves into the cultural, legal, and administrative challenges that arise, while providing coping strategies, resilience-building techniques, and information about support systems and resources available to help both parents and their adult children thrive despite the distance. "Roots Apart" is an indispensable resource for families facing the complexities of life when children settle abroad, offering guidance and reassurance for a fulfilling and connected future.

ABOUT THE AUTHOR

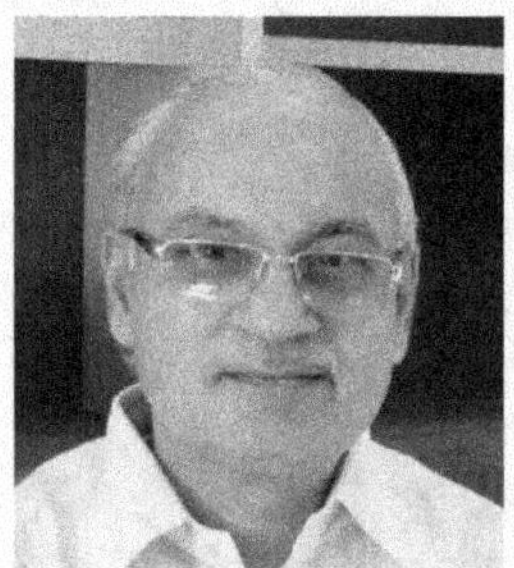

Mr. C. P. Kumar is a retired Scientist 'G' from National Institute of Hydrology, Roorkee, Uttarakhand, India. He is also a Reiki Healer and Chakra Balancing practitioner (with pendulum dowsing) and offers Emotional Freedom Technique (EFT) to help individuals with emotional issues. Mr. Kumar has authored many books on technical, spiritual, and social topics.

For further details, you may visit his webpage
https://www.angelfire.com/nh/cpkumar/virgo.html

www.ingramcontent.com/pod-product-compliance
Lightning Source LLC
Chambersburg PA
CBHW061519250726

48657CB00005B/1961